Do A 18O

JOIN THE
WELLNESS
REVOLUTION

Published by Advantage, Charleston, South Carolina.
Member of Advantage Media Group.

ADVANTAGE is a registered trademark, and the Advantage colophon is a trademark of Advantage Media Group, Inc.

Printed in the United States of America.

10 9 8 7 6 5 4

ISBN: 978-1-59932-875-1
LCCN: 2017941658

Book design by Lourn Eidal

Advantage Media Group is proud to be a part of the Tree Neutral® program. Tree Neutral offsets the number of trees consumed in the production and printing of this book by taking proactive steps such as planting trees in direct proportion to the number of trees used to print books. To learn more about Tree Neutral, please visit **www.treeneutral.com**.

Advantage Media Group is a publisher of business, self-improvement, and professional development books. We help entrepreneurs, business leaders, and professionals share their Stories, Passion, and Knowledge to help others Learn & Grow. Do you have a manuscript or book idea that you would like us to consider for publishing? Please visit advantagefamily.com or call **1.866.775.1696**.

This book is dedicated to Jeff Yates, my friend and brother in Christ, who decided to "Do a 180" and take charge of his health.

TABLE OF CONTENTS

Modern Medicine is Broken

You cannot trust conventional medicine and the pharmaceutical industry to enable you to obtain and maintain health.

The Pharmaceutical Medical Business Establishment controls medical care in the United States. This includes pharmaceutical, insurance and hospital corporations that have taken over medicine, forcing physicians and patients to follow their harmful protocols.

The various medical specialty societies have their lead physicians author clinical practice guidelines to influence the way physicians practice medicine. It has been published in the Journal of the American Medical Association (JAMA) that 87 percent of those physicians who author clinical practice guidelines have received financial support to perform research or have served as consultants or employees of the pharmaceutical companies.[1] This has the inevitable effect of creating biased clinical practice guidelines. This financial relationship represents a clear conflict of interest to any unbiased observer.

The Pharmaceutical Medical Business Establishment must be opposed and overturned.

A "Wellness Revolution" has begun among enlightened people and thinking physicians that will transform the way that individuals and medical professionals will approach health. It is exciting for me to have the opportunity to provide leadership in this "Wellness Revolution."

Dr. Benjamin Rush, signer of the Declaration of Independence, warned about the loss of medical freedom over 200 years ago. *"Unless we put medical freedom into the Constitution, the time will come when medicine will organize into an undercover dictatorship to restrict the art of healing to one class of Men and deny equal privileges to others; the Constitution of the Republic should make a Special privilege for medical freedoms as well as religious freedom."*

I would like to challenge you to join this "Wellness Revolution" and "Do a 180" and take charge of your health.

Those in the Pharmaceutical Medical Business Establishment support government controlled health care and the disease, drug and surgery model of medicine. They consider those who oppose them, to be medical heretics and disparage us because we have had the courage of our convictions to challenge their thinking and expose their corruption. Their opposition should be considered a red badge of honor.

I would like to challenge you to join this "Wellness Revolution" and "Do a 180" and take charge of your health.

There are millions of Americans and tens of thousands of physicians who support the "Wellness Revolution." They support free enterprise medical care and health savings accounts (HSA). They have abandoned the toxic approach of pharmaceutical drugs. They have adopted natural approaches to health. These patients have chosen to "Do a 180" and have taken charge of their health and these doctors have chosen to take charge of their medical practices. They are healthy and promoting natural approaches to health. They have permanently abandoned the dark side of medicine.

What I am going to be recommending for you to do is radical. It runs counter to the current conventional medical orthodoxy. In order for you to obtain and maintain your energy, vitality and health you will need to change the way you think and the way you live, and if you are a doctor, the way you operate your medical practice.

What I will be teaching you will be 180 degrees in the opposite direction to the way that "Big Pharma," the conventional medical establishment, the insurance companies, the hospital corporations and the federal government want you to think. This Pharmaceutical Medical Business Establishment views you as its cash cow. By keeping patients chronically sick, needing drugs, hospitalization and surgery, they have become its source of a recurring stream of income. There is no incentive for these business interests to promote natural, healthy measures to prevent the diseases associated with aging. Healthy people do not need their drugs nor services.

I have completely rejected that paradigm, that belief system, and have done a 180 from what I was taught to believe in medical school about the way to evaluate and treat my patients.

Unfortunately, the implicit message that I received during my medical education was that poor health was inevitable, and that, when it occurred, the solution was prescription drugs or surgery. I have completely rejected that paradigm, that belief system, and have done a 180 from what I was taught to believe in medical school about the way to evaluate and treat my patients.

Medical technology and surgical techniques in the United States are innovative and lead the rest of the world. If you have an acute health problem, such as a heart attack, a stroke or an accident, then the medical intervention that is required and the care that you receive from most medical doctors and at most large hospitals in our country, is world class. It is in treating the chronic problems that occur as we age, that conventional medicine falls short.

[1]Choudhry, NK, Stelfox, HT, and Detsky, A. Relationships between authors of clinical practice guidelines and the pharmaceutical idustr JAMA 2.6.2002; v287,S.

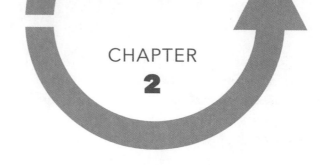

CHAPTER
2

Labelitis

Conventional medicine views various disturbed health conditions and symptoms, such as headaches, chronic fatigue syndrome, fibromyalgia, asthma, mood swings, insomnia, irritable bowel syndrome, gastroesophageal reflux, hypertension, Type 2 diabetes, coronary artery disease, cardiac arrhythmias, congestive heart disease, arthritis, and Alzheimer's disease as diagnoses. In reality, these are just symptoms that are given labels. This common disorder, known as *labelitis*, afflicts most doctors.

There is always an underlying cause, unfortunately most doctors are not taught to think about the cause or how to eliminate it.

Rather than trying to discover the underlying cause of the symptoms and establish a true diagnosis, conventional physicians will simply prescribe pharmaceutical drugs in an attempt to mask the symptoms. This is what their medical training has taught them to do. This is what I was taught to do.

According to Webster's dictionary, a *diagnosis* is the act of identifying the cause of a disease based upon the patient's signs and symptoms. Most conventional doctors rely primarily on blood tests. Webster's dictionary further explains that a *diagnosis* determines the underlying cause of a health condition or health problem. So, when your doctor tells you his diagnosis of your health problem, you should ask him, "Why do I have this problem?" There is always an underlying cause, unfortunately most doctors are not taught to think about the cause or how to eliminate it. They just mask your symptoms with drugs.

Conventional medicine attempts to understand these symptoms, which they incorrectly call diagnoses, based upon risk factors. If you were to ask your physician what causes heart attacks, his answer might be certain risk factors, such as elevated cholesterol, high blood pressure, type 2 diabetes, obesity, smoking, or stress. This still does not explain what caused the underlying risk factors or how poor lifestyle and eating habits create health problems.

Your doctor has been trained to prescribe a host of pharmaceutical drugs that not only will mask your symptoms, but will also cause a host of serious, adverse side effects.

> Your doctor has been trained to prescribe a host of pharmaceutical drugs that not only will mask your symptoms, but will also cause a host of serious, adverse side effects.

When your physician gives you these types of answers to your questions about high blood pressure, diabetes, heart attacks or any health problem, and wants to prescribe drugs for your symptoms, then you should keep asking him questions. Ask him what causes elevated cholesterol, elevated blood pressure, or type 2 diabetes. Ask him how poor lifestyle habits can cause you to develop health problems. Ask him why he thinks drugs are a solution to your health issues. Ask him about the dangerous side effects that are associated with the drugs that he wants to prescribe for you. Ask him whether there is a natural way to restore your health.

CHAPTER
3

Mitochondria, the Power Plants of Your Cells

Dr. Benjamin Rush, a Founding Father of the United States, expressed his Unifying Principle of Disease in 1796. *"The multiplication of diseases is as repugnant to truth in medicine, as polytheism is to truth in religion. The physician who considers every different affection of the different systems of the body as distinct diseases when they arise from one cause, resembles the Indian or African savage, who considers water, dew, ice, frost and snow as distinct essences."* Dr. Rush realized that there were many medical problems, but there was only one single, unifying cause. Modern science has discovered this cause.

Diseases are caused by low energy production in your cells. The primary reason that you may suffer from heart and other health problems as you mature is because the *power plants* within your cells, known as *mitochondria*, lack the ability to produce adequate amounts of energy necessary for the organs of your body to function optimally.

> Diseases are caused by low energy production in your cells.

This decline in energy production is caused by toxins in the environment, specifically, chemicals found in the air you breathe, the foods and drinks you consume and the lotions you apply to your skin. Heavy metals, such as mercury, lead and aluminum, recurrent infections, including dental and gum disease, as well as a high sugar, simple carbohydrate diet are all

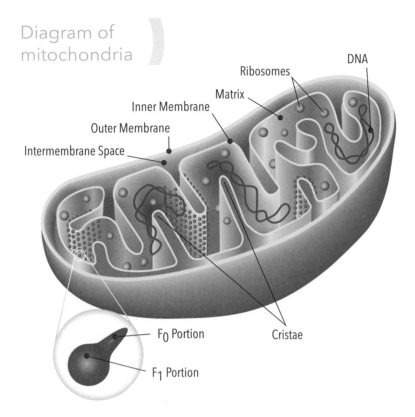

Diagram of
mitochondria

DNA

Ribosomes

Matrix

Inner Membrane

Outer Membrane

Intermembrane Space

F_0 Portion

Cristae

F_1 Portion

culprits. This energy decline may also be due to the lack of the proper vitamins, minerals, nutrients and hormones required by the mitochondria in your cells to produce optimal energy levels necessary for healthy functioning of the cells and organs. Lack of exercise also contributes to low energy production.

When your cells are toxic, the mitochondria cannot produce adequate amounts of energy. This means that your cells will be sick, which makes your organs and your whole body sick, producing numerous symptoms and the medical conditions that were previously mentioned. Seeking relief from your symptoms, you visit your physician for evaluation and treatment. After drawing a few blood tests and performing a brief history and physical exam, he will invariably prescribe some pharmaceutical drugs as Band-Aids to mask your symptoms. Because all drugs are toxins, this just adds to the toxic load in your cells and makes you sicker, quicker.

Nobody is sick because they have low levels of pharmaceutical drugs in their body. These drugs are all toxins. During my first semester in medical school, I took a course in pharmacology. One of the chapters in the pharmacology textbook discussed the detoxification of drugs. Drugs have to be detoxified by the liver. In Webster's dictionary, the first definition of toxin is poison. This means that the drugs that your physician prescribes to you are poisons. That's right, they are poisons. This is why they cause the numerous harmful side effects which are described to you when you watch a pharmaceutical drug's advertisement on television.

> Nobody is sick because they have low levels of pharmaceutical drugs in their body.

If you come away from reading this book with only the realization that all pharmaceutical drugs are poisons, that they poison your cells and make you sicker quicker, and that their long-term use should be avoided like the plague, then I will feel like I have been successful. **You must now decide whether you are ready to "Do a 180" and take charge of your health.**

You do not have to be a rocket scientist to know that you cannot poison yourself to good health. This is just good, old-fashioned common sense and there has never been an epidemic of common sense, especially in the medical profession.

CHAPTER
4

My Personal "180"

My dad had great common sense. The best advice he ever gave me was when, on the night of my graduation from medical school in July, 1976, he told me, "Son, don't poison your patients like all the other doctors do." This seed that he planted in my mind on my graduation night, took firm root and has grown into a mighty oak that has produced a passion in me for developing natural approaches to health and wellness and to develop the Hotze Health & Wellness Center and its allied businesses, Hotze Vitamins and Hotze Pharmacy.

> ❝ Son, don't poison your patients like all the other doctors do."

Thank you Dad.

The following discussion will explain the thought process that led me to my conclusion that the current conventional medicine model that labels symptoms as diseases and then prescribes drugs to mask those symptoms, is outdated and equivalent to believing that the world is flat. This medical paradigm must be repudiated.

My Mom and Dad taught me to question conventional thinking and not simply accept the status quo.

My father, Ernest Hotze, was an engineer who rose to become vice president of sales for Dresser Clark. He later went on to establish his own business, Compressor Engineering Corporation (CECO). Dad was an outstanding salesman and entrepreneur.

With seven sons and one daughter, he had to be. Dad instilled in us a desire to excel beyond the norm and hold ourselves to high standards.

My mother, Margaret, who earned a journalism degree from the University of Texas, was a voracious reader. She constantly challenged me to "break out of the box" and question conventional thought. If she told me once, then she told me scores of times, **"Never follow the crowd because it is usually going in the wrong direction. Move away from the crowd and lead it in the right direction."**

During my years at St. Thomas High School, an all-boys' Catholic school in Houston, I took her leadership advice to heart. There, I played quarterback on the football team and was elected student body president. Nothing was more exhilarating to me than getting into a tight situation, pulling the team together in a huddle, and calling the play. The football coaches at St. Thomas reinforced the values that I had received at home, challenging me to excel. Though we played many of the top-ranked public high schools, every time we set foot on the field we fully expected to win, and win we did.

> My experiences have taught me that with every adversity there is a seed of equal or greater opportunity in the future.

We played in the Texas Catholic Interscholastic State Championship every year I was in high school and won the state title three out of four years.

The winning spirit instilled in me by my parents and my coaches has produced in me a steel-willed determination to overcome obstacles in order to achieve my goals. My experiences have taught me that with every adversity there is a seed of equal or greater opportunity in the future.

Football also brought my wife of forty-eight years into my life. Janie, who attended Duchesne Academy, an all-girls' school, was one of our varsity cheerleaders. During the summer after our senior year in high school, Janie and I eloped to Mexico. I do not think this is what my mother had in mind when she advised me not to follow the crowd. My father told me that I had made my bed and I was going to have to sleep in it. With seven other children, he was in no position to help us financially, nor did we expect that of him.

Janie and I moved to Austin, Texas, so that I could attend college. Janie worked for the first two years of our marriage, until the birth of our second child, while I attended the University of Texas and set up a paint contracting and remodeling business. Even though I was working, I managed to graduate from college in three and a half years. Little did I know that my real education was only about to begin. I was accepted into medical school.

> After years of thinking outside the box, I found myself in an environment where questioning the status quo was not encouraged.

In 1972, I entered the University of Texas Medical School at Houston. The first two years consisted solely of classroom lectures and laboratory work. The final two years were clinical rotations in internal medicine, obstetrics and gynecology, psychiatry, pediatrics, cardiology, surgery, and other specialties.

Medical school required some adjustment. After years of thinking outside the box, I found myself in an environment where questioning the status quo was not encouraged. The young doctors-to-be were expected to receive instruction from their elders, not question it. This didn't come naturally to me.

My psychiatry rotation proved to be my most difficult. Most of the patients in the psychiatric wards of the hospital were taking mind-altering medications such as antidepressants, antipsychotics, and tranquilizers. Their faces were expressionless, with emptiness in their eyes. They walked in a jerky manner and made rolling motions with their fingers. These were the side effects of the powerful drugs that they had been prescribed.

During my psychiatry rotation, I also observed patients with depression undergoing electroshock therapy. The doctor would place paddles on each side of the patient's head and administer currents of electricity. When the patients were shocked, their bodies would become rigid and undergo seizure-like activity. Because the electric shock to the brain would destroy memory, patients often remained depressed after this therapy but did not remember why. The treatment was barbaric and should be banned.

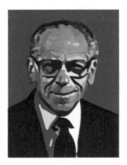

Dr. Thomas Szasz
1920-2012

During my psychiatric rotation, I read a book called *The Myth of Mental Illness*, by Dr. Tom Szasz, a prominent psychiatrist. In this book, he criticized what he called the "psycho-babble" of modern-day psychiatry and its attempt to redefine psychological problems as medical diseases. By classifying peculiarities of thinking or behavior as diseases, he charged that psychiatry had absolved individuals of responsibility for their actions. The drug companies capitalized on this by synthesizing a host of psychiatric medications to "treat" these new diseases.

Dr. Szasz's arguments impressed me. Unfortunately, my professors did not share my point of view and gave me an F at the end of my psychiatry rotation. I was required to retake psychiatry the spring of my fourth year in medical school. Since passing this clinical rotation was a requirement of graduation, I decided that discretion was the better part of valor. So the second time around, I spouted back exactly what my psychiatry professors wanted to hear and earned a passing grade.

It was during my surgical rotation that I was taught the surgeons' motto: "A chance to cut is a chance to cure." The surgeons I encountered tended to frown upon the use of drugs, recognizing— quite rightly—that drugs do not cure disease but merely alleviate symptoms. However, the surgeons simply replaced one technique for managing symptoms with a more extreme one: cutting or removing the organ in which the symptoms were manifested. Of course, many of these surgical interventions were necessary, but could have been prevented had the patients been instructed on how to obtain and maintain health and wellness, naturally.

> The surgeons' motto: "A chance to cut is a chance to cure."

During my surgical rotation, I witnessed this drastic approach to symptom management countless times. For example, hysterectomies were routinely recommended when women experienced heavy menstrual bleeding and cramps. The surgeons performing these operations believed that removing the target organ, the uterus, would cure the problem. Well, yes, without a uterus a woman will no longer experience heavy periods and breakthrough bleeding. But what if the uterus was not the cause of the problem? More important, what if the underlying cause could be identified and corrected? If this was possible, then millions of women could be spared the ordeal of surgery and the host of problems resulting from removal of the uterus and ovaries.

These were not questions I felt prepared to ask at this early stage in my medical career. Soon, though, I would meet a mentor who would encourage me to ask them. This would lead to my personal "180."

CHAPTER
5

Learning to Ask "Why?"

In 1976, I graduated from the University of Texas medical school at Houston, passed the state boards, and received my medical license. That fall, I began my surgical internship at St. Joseph's Hospital in Houston.

During my internship I was fortunate to work under a remarkable physician, Dr. Herb Fred, who was the Director of Postgraduate Education at St. Joseph's Hospital. He was a brilliant clinician who was able to see the big picture. He taught the newly minted doctors the necessity of making our diagnoses based upon the clinical history and physical examination of our patients, rather than by relying strictly upon laboratory tests.

> Dr. Fred was emphatic in his message that we would never become excellent physicians unless we learned to ask "Why?"

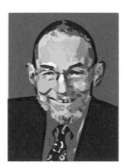

Dr. Herb Fred

Dr. Fred used the Socratic method of teaching. When we presented patient cases with our diagnoses to Dr. Fred, he would always ask us, "Why is that so?" We would respond, and he would again ask, "Well, why is that so?" This dialogue would continue until he had exposed our ignorance and demonstrated that, in fact, we did not know why it was so.

Dr. Fred was emphatic in his message that we would never become excellent physicians unless we learned to ask "Why?" "Why does this patient have recurrent infections?

Why does this patient have headaches? Why is this patient fatigued or depressed? Why does this patient have high blood pressure? Why does this patient have diabetes? Why does this patient have asthma? Why does this patient have heart disease? Why? Why? Why?" In short, what is the underlying cause of the patient's symptoms? As a corollary to that, why should I believe that drugs, with their numerous side effects, would resolve this patient's problems? Could there be a safer, more natural way to address the underlying cause?

Dr. Fred would chastise us by saying, "The problem with you and most people is that you are not willing to think and ask 'why?'. The reason for this is that thinking takes time and it is hard, and you are lazy."

> **"Why? Why? Why?"** In short, what is the underlying cause of the patient's symptoms?

Unfortunately, there are not many professors like Dr. Fred who challenge their students to question conventional thinking. Dr. Fred's teaching has had a profound influence on my approach to medicine.

Whenever one of my patients has not improved on my recommended treatment plan, I ask myself, "Why isn't this patient getting better? What else could be going on? What other natural approaches could be offered that would resolve this problem?"

This type of questioning, when determining the true cause of a person's medical problems, has enabled me to provide natural solutions that have yielded remarkable results in the lives of tens of thousands of our guests at the Hotze Health & Wellness Center. Asking questions, listening to our guest's answers, and documenting their reported improvements is what has allowed me to develop my current treatment program.

CHAPTER
6

Helping Guests To "Do A 180"

We decided to enter the hospitality industry, benchmarking with The Ritz-Carlton and The Broadmoor in Colorado Springs, and within that context, provide medical care.

You may find it odd that I refer to our patients as guests. In 1997, the President of my company, Monica Luedecke, and I decided we no longer wanted to be solely in the practice of medicine. Most medical practices are terrible failures when it comes to customer service. Any restaurant that provided customer service on par with most medical practices would have been out of business within a month. Instead, we decided to enter the hospitality industry, benchmarking with The Ritz-Carlton and The Broadmoor in Colorado Springs, and within that context, provide medical care. At the time, this was a revolutionary concept. I was even chastised by one of the members of the Texas Medical Board for referring to our patients as "guests." I believe that the way we treat our guests is as important, if not more important, than the treatment we prescribe. People who seek medical care want to feel listened to, understood, affirmed and given hope that their health can be restored. This is what we have been practicing at the Hotze Health & Wellness Center since 1989.

Our **Growth Vision Statement** at the Hotze Health & Wellness Center reads,

"Our purpose is to enable our guests to enjoy a better quality of life by helping them obtain and maintain health and wellness, naturally. Our growth rests upon the foundation of extraordinary hospitality and guest experiences. We are building the finest health and wellness business in the world. We are leading a 'Wellness Revolution' which will change the way women and men are treated through detoxification and bioidentical hormone replacement. Our vision for the future differentiates us from our competitors. We commit to increase our knowledge and skills, individually and as a team, to ensure that we achieve our goals."

Our **Mission Statement** at the Hotze Health & Wellness Center reads,

"We are committed to helping you to obtain and maintain health and wellness, naturally, so that you enjoy a better quality of life. This goal can be achieved by increasing your energy level and strengthening your immune system."

Let me give you an example of the common presentation that we see in many of our guests. They present with fatigue, weight gain, high blood pressure, insomnia, brain fog, mood swings, joint and muscle aches and pains, gastroesophageal reflux,

> The medications that were prescribed to them simply added fuel to the fire, making them more toxic.

menstrual irregularities, allergies, leading to recurrent sinus and bronchial infections, headaches, adult onset diabetes, among other symptoms. They have often seen numerous conventional physicians who had simply tried to treat their symptoms by prescribing various pharmaceutical drugs, such as high blood pressure medication, anti-inflammatories, statin drugs to lower cholesterol, the "purple pill," Nexium, for reflux, anti-diabetic drugs, antidepressants, anti-anxiety and sleep medications, to name a few. The reason these individuals had their symptoms to begin with was because their cells were toxic and their mitochondria, the power plants within their cells, were producing low levels of energy. Now, the medications that were prescribed to them simply added fuel to the fire, making them more toxic.

It is always our goal to get our guests off these pharmaceutical medications as soon as possible. Some drugs can be stopped immediately, such as the anti-inflammatories and statin drugs, as well as medication for gastroesophageal reflux. Other drugs, such as high blood pressure and antidepressant medications, must be weaned over time as the individual begins to experience a positive response to treatment of yeast and a paleo eating lifestyle, hormonal replenishment, vitamin and mineral supplementation, and the adoption of an exercise program.

> It is always our goal to get our guests off these pharmaceutical medications as soon as possible.

For most of our guests, this approach has turned out to be a godsend. Their blood pressure normalizes on magnesium and potassium supplementation, allowing them to eliminate their blood pressure medications. Magnesium and potassium deficiency is often the root cause of their high blood pressure. Their muscle aches and pains diminish once the toxic effects of the statin drugs wear off. Their reflux is eliminated on the yeast free, Paleo eating lifestyle. Their overall energy levels are restored once the mitochondria in their cells begin to produce more energy as a result of thyroid and other hormone replenishment and vitamin and mineral supplementation.

When your cells are toxic, they produce low levels of energy, making you sick. When your cells produce high levels of energy, then you will be healthy.

At the Hotze Health & Wellness Center, we have evaluated and treated over 30,000 guests over the past 27 years, beginning in 1989. This brief explanation of our evaluation and treatment program is how we have approached solving our guests' health issues. If this approach had not worked, then I would have continued to ask myself the question, "Why?" Because it has worked in the vast majority of our guests who stay on the program, I commonly have them tell me, "Thank you for giving me back my life!" or "You saved my life."

> If this approach had not worked, then I would have continued to ask myself the question, "Why?"

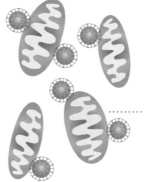

TOXIC CELLS

HEALTHY CELLS

This is the reason that I am leading a "Wellness Revolution," encouraging physicians, you and other individuals, to "Do a 180," take charge of your health, and join this "Wellness Revolution." When you do, you will begin to experience an exceptional, enthusiastic life, full of vitality and energy.

Your life depends upon it.

ABOUT THE AUTHOR

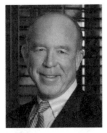

STEVEN F. HOTZE, MD
Author, Founder and Chief Executive Officer of Hotze Enterprises

Steven F. Hotze, MD, is the founder and CEO of the Hotze Health & Wellness Center, Hotze Vitamins and Hotze Pharmacy. Dr. Hotze is leading a "Wellness Revolution!" His goal is to change the way women and men are treated in midlife through the use of bioidentical hormone therapy. Since 1989, his 8-Point Treatment Regimen has helped over 30,000 individuals to get on a path of health and wellness and enjoy a better quality of life in an environment of extraordinary hospitality and guest service.

Dr. Hotze is the author of the books, *Hormones, Health, and Happiness* and *Hypothyroidism, Health & Happiness*. In these, he describes his journey from using pharmaceutical drugs to actively listening to his patients and treating the root cause of their symptoms through natural approaches. "For an acute illness, such as strep throat or a sinus infection, the drug approach may be appropriate. However, few patients with chronic ailments ever really get well by taking drugs. How can they? Chronic illness and disease are not caused by deficiencies of prescription drugs."

Suzanne Somers dedicated an entire chapter to Dr. Hotze in her *New York Times* best seller, *Breakthrough*. "This Texan doctor is going to steal your heart," writes Somers. "He has so much energy he can't wait to get to his office each day. He has built up a practice that is the envy of doctors everywhere."

Dr. Hotze has appeared on hundreds of television and radio shows across the nation, including ABC, NBC, CBS, and FOX affiliates, and CBS' The Morning Show. He has also appeared nationally on CNN. He is also a regular guest on the KHOU Channel 11 morning program, Great Day Houston and hosts his own radio program, "Dr. Hotze's Wellness Revolution" weekdays from 1 – 2 pm on KPRC AM 950 in Houston.

Dr. Hotze is a member of the the Association of American Physicians and Surgeons. He is a past president of the Pan American Allergy Society, and is a current member of the board of directors. He earned his medical degree from University of Texas at Houston in 1976.

Dr. Hotze and his wife, Janie, have been married for 48 years and are the parents of eight children and twenty-two grandchildren to date.

Steven F. Hotze, M.D.
Founder and CEO – Hotze Health & Wellness Center
www.hotzehwc.com
www.DoA180.com
www.menshealthandenergy.org
www.drhotze.com

Contact information:
Phone: 281.698.8698
Email: info@drhotze.com